READY TO

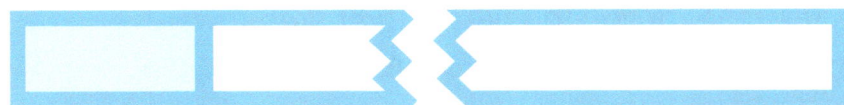

QUIT

making your plan to
become a nonsmoker

This book is only to help you learn. It
should not be used to replace any advice
or treatment from your health care provider.

Facing the challenge

Forty-three million people have quit smoking, and you can too. That's about half of all living adults who have ever smoked! These new nonsmokers have found healthier, happier lives free from the dangers of nicotine. You deserve the same chance.

Now is the time for you to take the first step toward quitting. Don't worry if you have already tried to quit before. Each try improves your chance of quitting for good. Most former smokers tried more than once to quit.

> Take the first brave step toward freedom. Imagine yourself as a nonsmoker.

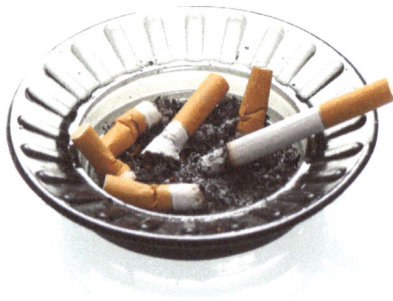

You didn't decide to get hooked on smoking, but you can decide to quit. Maybe you haven't made up your mind. Can you imagine your life if you didn't have to smoke?

> Smoking is the largest single preventable cause of death and disability in America.

Where am I?

Check the most honest statement about how you feel right now.

- ☐ I am not planning to quit smoking at this time.

- ☐ I am seriously thinking about quitting in the next 6 months.

- ☐ I am ready to quit, and I intend to quit within the next 30 days.

- ☐ I have just quit (within the last 6 months), and I need help.

- ☐ It has been 6 months to a year since I quit, and I don't want to start back.

- ☐ I just relapsed and I want to quit again.

Many people change their minds a number of times before they are ready to take action.

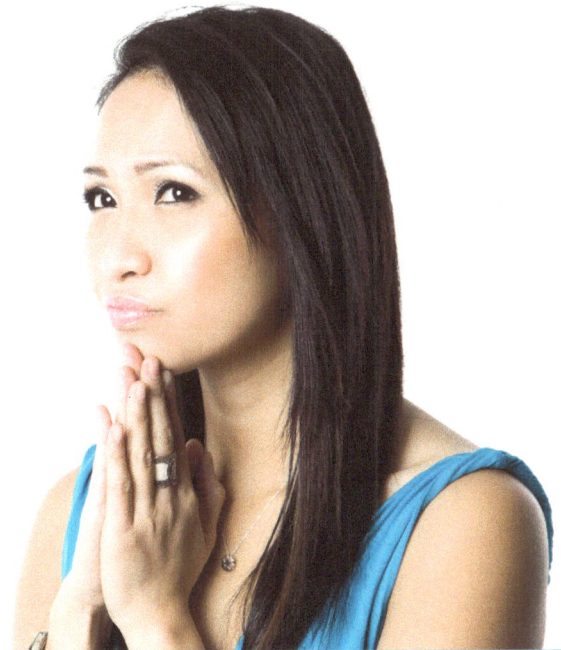

> Be honest about how you feel, and be willing to learn.

These stages are adapted from the work of Dr. J.O. Prochaska, University of Rhode Island.

Why don't I want to quit?

"I feel too much stress to even think about quitting."

Almost everyone has felt stress at one time or another. When you use cigarettes to help you deal with stress, your body reacts by increasing your heart rate and blood pressure. This may make you feel even more stressed. There are many other ways to deal with stress that are much more healthy for you. (See pages 13 and 14.)

"I will gain too much weight when I quit."

Though some people gain weight, you don't have to lose control of your weight to quit smoking. On average, a person who quits smoking gains about 5 pounds. One in 5 people who quit smoking gain no weight at all. Plan to exercise as you quit. This will help prevent weight gain.

"It's too late. The damage is done."

Not true! Even if you now smoke a pack a day, your extra risk for heart disease is cut in half the first year after quitting. After 10 years, your risk for mouth, throat and other cancers will have dropped by half.* If you have already had a heart attack, quitting will reduce your chances of having another heart attack. It's never too late to quit!

* American Cancer Society - Benefits of Quitting Smoking Over Time

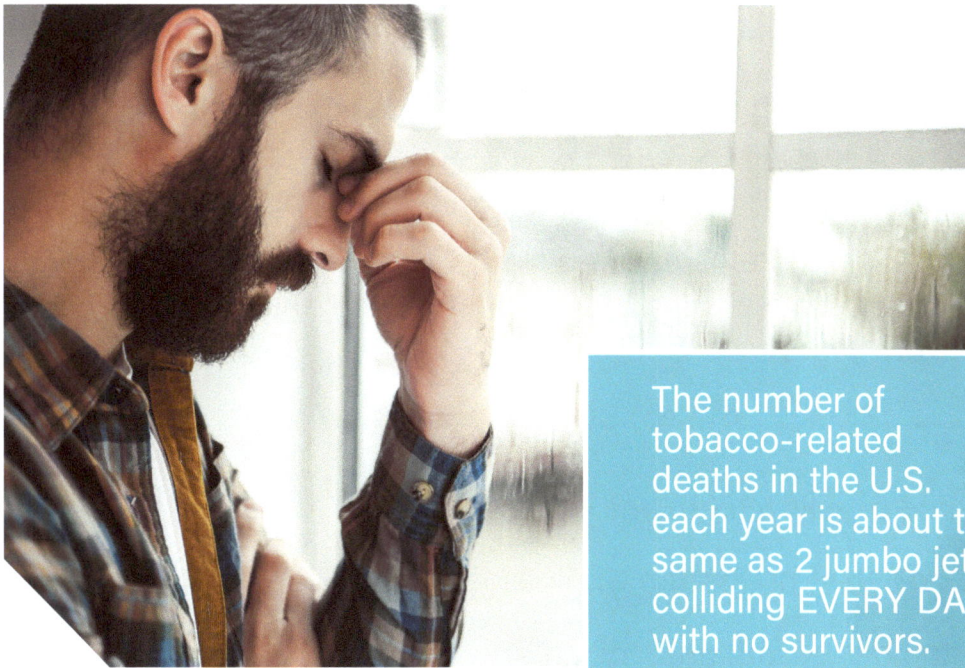

The number of tobacco-related deaths in the U.S. each year is about the same as 2 jumbo jets colliding EVERY DAY with no survivors.

"Everybody is going to die sometime. I'll take my chances."

Why gamble with your life? You stack the odds in your favor when you quit smoking. The people who love you want you to stick around.

"Nobody tells me what to do. I have a right to smoke."

No one likes to be controlled. But when you think about it, aren't you being controlled by your habit? And the chronic illness from smoking can control your whole life.

"I'm not hurting anyone but me."

Wrong. Secondhand smoke can cause breathing and heart problems in your family and friends. Children who live in a house with a smoker are more likely to get asthmatic bronchitis, middle ear infections and even pneumonia. Smoking in another room is not enough to protect them.

Why do I want to quit?

Check all of the items that you really care about. Do not mark items just because you think you should care about them. These are your reasons.

Personal reasons

- ☐ tired of yellow teeth and fingers
- ☐ don't want premature wrinkles
- ☐ stop bad breath and dry mouth
- ☐ want food to taste better
- ☐ don't want gum disease and tooth loss
- ☐ tired of smelly clothes, smelly house, smelly car
- ☐ want to spend less time cleaning dirty walls, windows, mirrors
- ☐ no more messy ashtrays
- ☐ no more smoker's cough
- ☐ to have two free hands
- ☐ take charge of my life again
- ☐ feel better about myself
- ☐ make my family proud
- ☐ stop being a fire hazard
- ☐ tired of being treated like a second-class citizen
- ☐ no more panic at getting caught in no smoking areas
- ☐ look forward to an active retirement

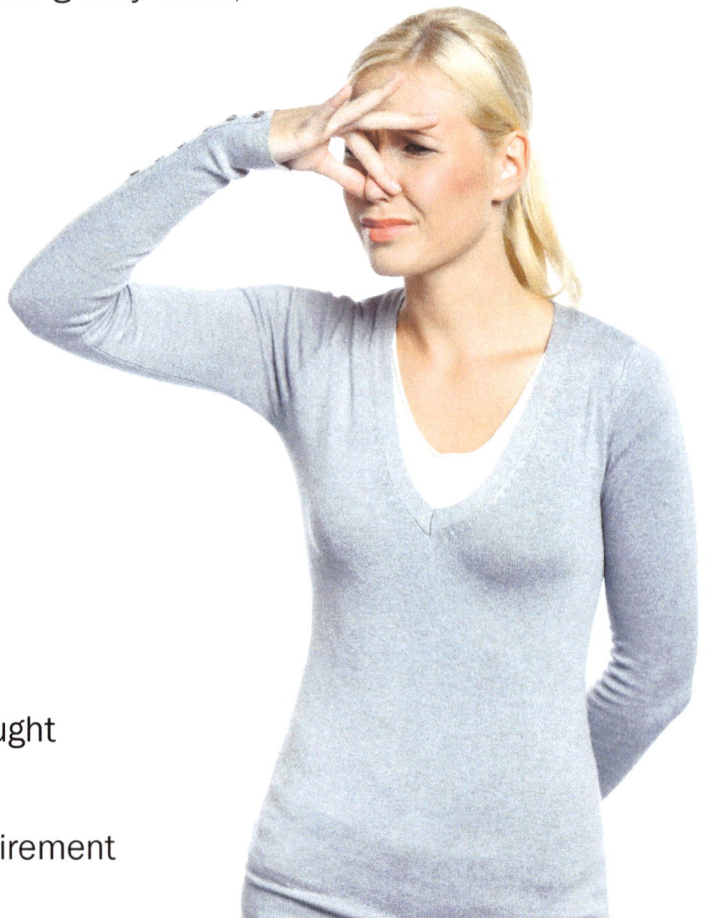

Financial reasons

- ☐ save $_____a year (cost of a pack of cigarettes x number of packs you smoke a day x 365 days = savings in one year)

- ☐ want lower (nonsmoker) insurance rates

- ☐ fewer sick days for smoke-related illness

- ☐ fewer days staying home with sick child

- ☐ want to spend retirement money on travel, not medical bills

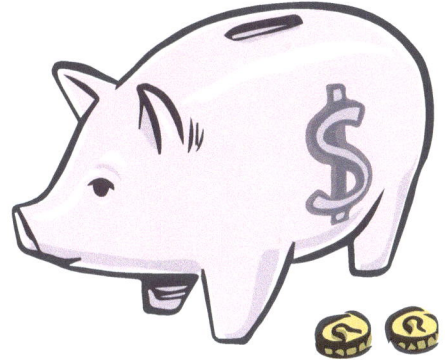

Health reasons

- ☐ want to breathe easier

- ☐ want more energy and endurance

- ☐ improve circulation to whole body

- ☐ reduce allergies and sinus problems

- ☐ reduce bouts of chronic bronchitis

- ☐ want to lower my risk for heart attack or stroke

- ☐ don't want to be short-winded from emphysema

- ☐ reduce my risk of lung cancer

- ☐ help avoid bladder and kidney cancer

- ☐ help avoid cancer of mouth, throat or voice box

- ☐ reduce chances for cancer of pancreas

- ☐ help my stomach ulcers heal

- ☐ reduce number of asthma attacks

- ☐ improve chances of surviving another heart attack

- ☐ recover faster from surgery

Example:

$7.00 a pack x 3 packs a day

x 365 days a year

―――――――――――――

= $7,665 saved per year

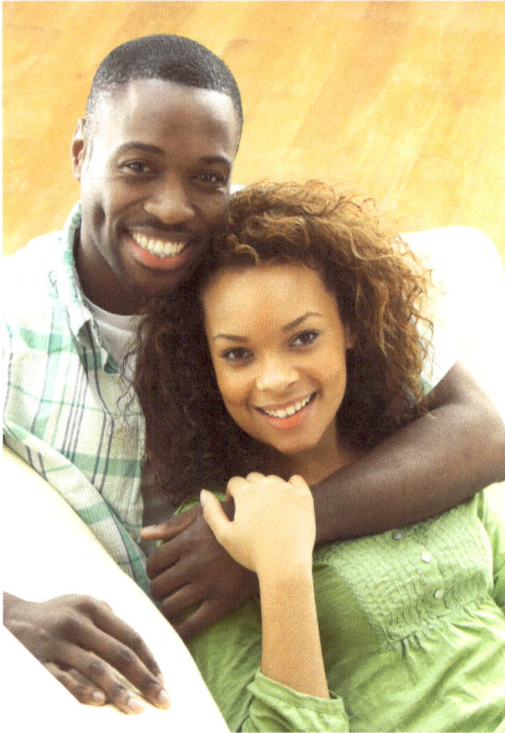

Family reasons

- ☐ make my family happy

- ☐ want to live to see my grandchildren grow up

- ☐ spend more time with my family, not outside smoking

- ☐ stop exposing them to nasty odors

- ☐ don't want to help cause breathing problems and other health problems to my family

- ☐ be a better role model

- ☐ don't want my children to suffer from ear infections, asthma or pneumonia

Women's issues

- ☐ tired of coughing so hard—it makes me leak urine

- ☐ want the option to take birth control pills, which I might not be able to do if I smoke

- ☐ don't want to be 10 times more likely to miscarry

- ☐ want to have a normal birth weight baby

- ☐ don't want my baby to have 3 times greater chance of birth defects

- ☐ don't want 50% greater chance of infant crib death for my children

Other reasons

Why I smoke

Now that you have decided on some good reasons to quit, it's time to check out the reasons you smoke. This section will help you understand what you get out of smoking cigarettes so you can meet those needs in a healthier way.

Your plan for quitting will work better if you include lots of substitutes for smoking needs. The next few pages will give you some ideas for how to do this.

I smoke for energy

Smoking meets your need for a "pick-me-up." You need new ways to get you going in the morning and to give you a boost throughout the day. When you get up in the morning, don't have a cigarette. Instead:

- turn on lots of lights

- use an intense mouthwash

- put on some lively music

- do some stretching exercises

- sing loudly in the shower

- drink your coffee on the porch

Throughout the day, take stretch, exercise or singing breaks. If you can't take a break, just hum or whistle.

Make a list of some more "pick-me-ups" that you might try:

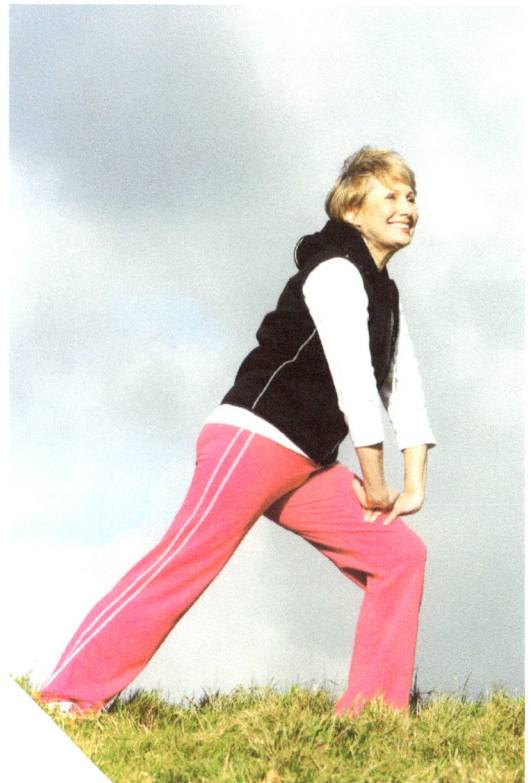

Make a plan to keep mind and body busy. Regular exercise is the best way to keep your body and mind sharp and alert. Build up to at least 30 minutes of exercise, most days of the week. Choose something that fits your interests, lifestyle and state of health. **Always ask your doctor before starting any exercise program.**

You might try one or more of these:

- walking
- jogging
- yoga
- biking
- swimming
- dancing

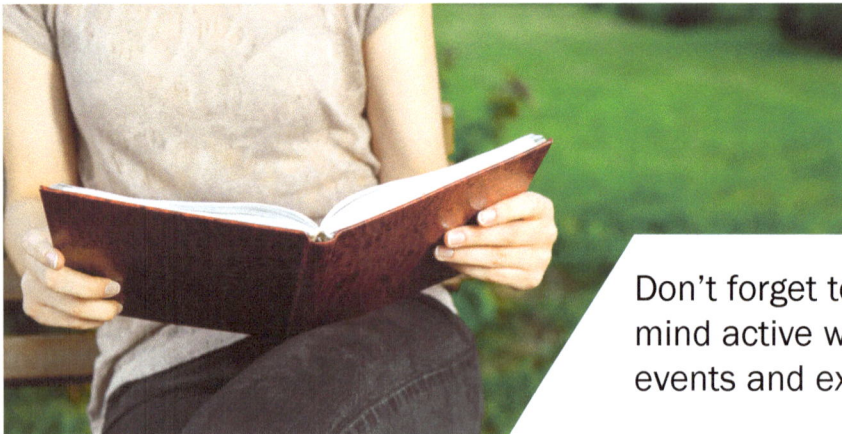

Don't forget to keep your mind active with fun events and exciting goals:

- read a good book
- take music lessons
- start a garden
- join a card club
- go to a play, movie or concert
- volunteer
- take a class in cooking, drawing, painting, pottery, woodworking, etc.

Write down some other things you might like to do to keep your body and mind active:

I like the feel of smoking and holding a cigarette

Your plan should include other ways to keep your hands busy. Try these:

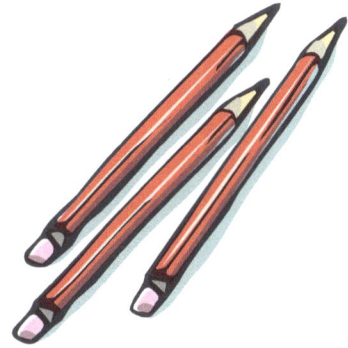

- pen
- pencil
- sponge ball
- worry stone

- heavy coin
- rubber band
- paper clip
- hard candy

- sugar-free gum
- carrot or celery sticks
- straw
- cinnamon stick

You will be surprised at how it helps to play with a rubber band or chew gum when you're a "handler."

When you're at home, you can put together jigsaw puzzles, models or picture albums. When the urge to smoke is very strong, get busy using both hands. Do things like dry dishes, polish silver, weed the garden or carve wood.

Be creative with your "handiness." Have fun learning card or coin tricks and other sleights of hand. You could knit, sew or crochet. Keep a crossword puzzle or doodle pad handy. Make a list of other things you could do that would keep your hands busy and that you would enjoy:

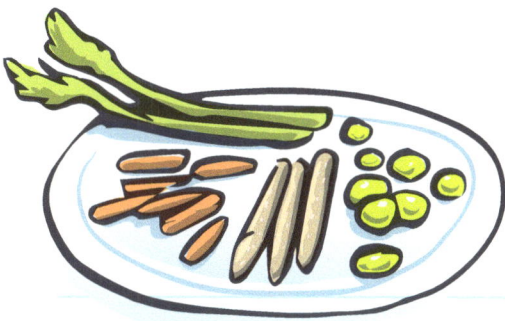

> If you are a nibbler, stock your kitchen with low calorie snacks like carrot sticks, celery, crunchy bread sticks and grapes.

I smoke to relax and feel good

Smoking can feel like a reward sometimes. You may find it hard to relax without smoking. Instead of smoking, treat yourself to **lots of little pleasures and big rewards.** What do you love to do?

- Schedule time to read or to just do nothing.

- Spend some fun time with your family or friends or quiet time by yourself.

- Give yourself a night off from the usual chores.

- Treat yourself to a manicure, pedicure, new hairdo or makeover.

- Buy the hobby supplies you need with the money you used to spend on cigarettes.

- Get a massage.

- Go to some of the movies, plays and concerts you've been wanting to see.

- Go to dinner with the funniest people you know.

- Play sports that you like. Do exercises that you enjoy.

Make a list of some of your favorite rewards:

Instead of lighting up a cigarette when you get home from work, change into your favorite "at home" clothes to mark the start of your free time. Sit down with your favorite magazine for a while. Lie in the hammock. Relax with a soak in a warm tub.

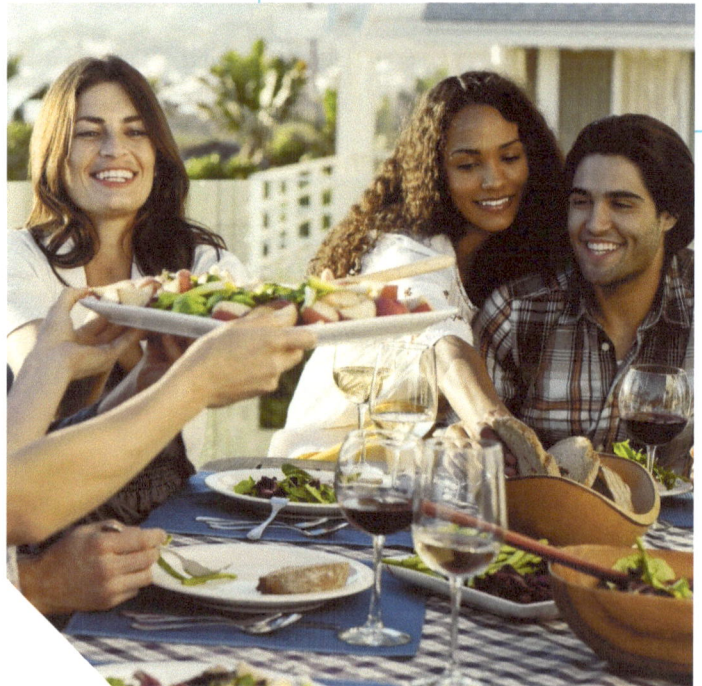

I smoke for stress relief

If you light up when you are angry, upset or blue, you don't smoke to feel good, you smoke to avoid feeling bad. **It takes courage to handle your feelings in other ways.** It may help to talk to someone.

If you can't talk to someone when you are upset, here are some other ways to blow off steam. Keep in mind that the urge to smoke will pass even if you don't act on it.

- "Mash" a squeeze toy.
- Play a sound-effects toy.
- Chop vegetables.
- Do a hammer and nail project.

- Sing as loudly as you can.
- Chop wood.
- Do an aerobic exercise.
- Take a warm bath or shower.

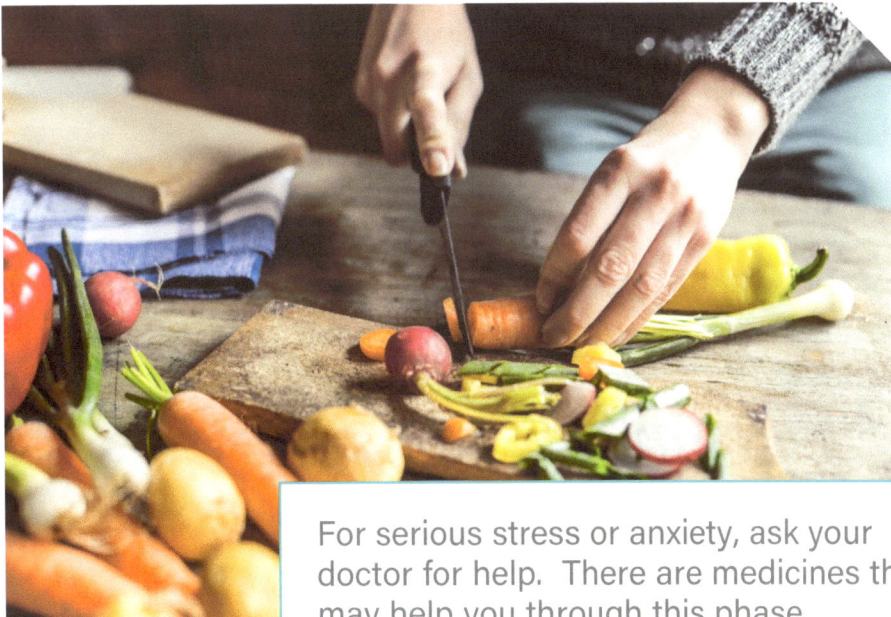

For serious stress or anxiety, ask your doctor for help. There are medicines that may help you through this phase.

chronic stress

Chronic stress occurs when you have more problems in your life than you can control. You can find relief by getting rid of some problems and by learning how to relax.

Stressors can be workload, physical problems, abusive people, lack of sleep, debt, trying to do too much, etc. Straight talk and setting healthy limits will allow you to take better care of yourself. Ask your doctor or someone from your employee assistance program to recommend a counselor if you find you can't make these changes on your own.

Active exercise is very good after tedious (or boring) stress such as office work, assembly lines, travel, waiting, long meetings or lectures. Some active exercises include housework, yard work, walking or aerobic workouts.

Relaxation exercises are great for stressful times such as deadlines, tight schedules and noisy children. Some relaxation exercises include meditation, deep breathing, muscle relaxation and massage.

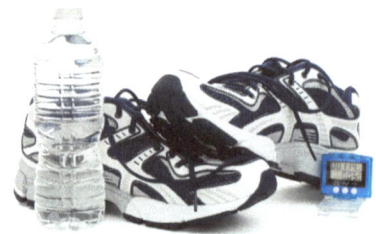

The best stress reducer is free, healthy and needs no prescription. It's EXERCISE!

A Simple Relaxation Exercise:

1. Find a comfortable spot and close your eyes.

2. Concentrate on breathing from your stomach without raising your shoulders.

3. Each time you exhale, let a little more tension drain out of your body.

4. Allow your shoulders to sink and your jaw to drop a little.

5. Imagine that your body is disappearing.

6. Pretend you are reappearing in a pleasant memory or a new fantasy. Let yourself stay in that calm scene as long as you can.

I smoke because I'm hooked

If you:

- **panic** when you are out of cigarettes

- **think about smoking** even when you aren't smoking

- **have a real hunger for a smoke** when you haven't had one for a while. Then you most likely have a physical addiction.

If you are addicted, you can expect some or all of these withdrawal symptoms when you try to quit:

- anxiety, irritability

- trouble concentrating

- urges to smoke

- frustration, anger

- increased appetite

- depression

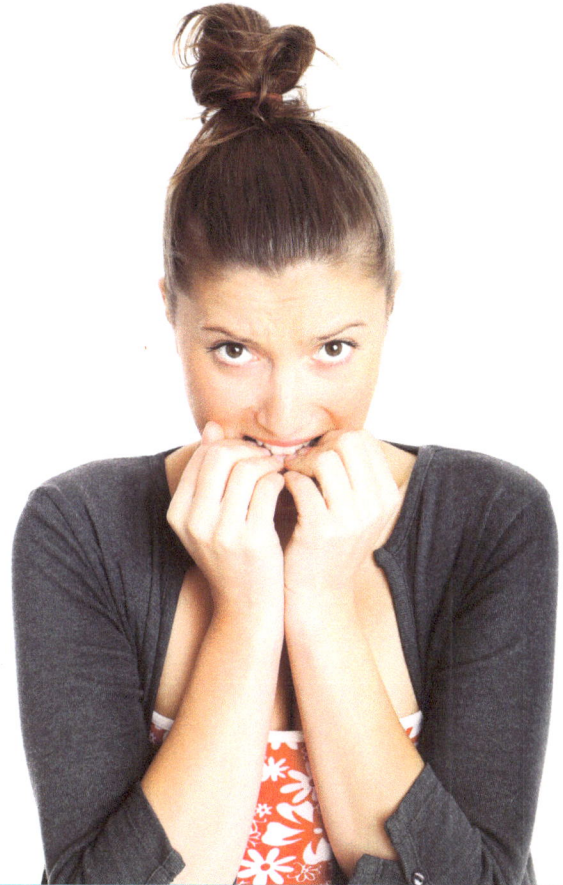

Limit your use of coffee and alcohol when you first quit smoking. Caffeine can cause you to be nervous and to have trouble sleeping. Alcohol lowers your self-control and makes it easier to slip. Stay hydrated by drinking water (if your doctor says it's ok.)

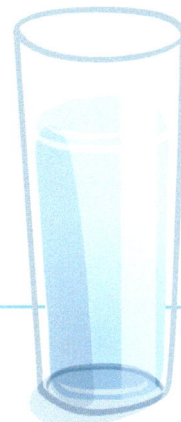

I smoke and don't know I'm smoking

If you smoke without:

- being aware of it

- knowing you have a cigarette burning in an ashtray

- remembering you even put the cigarette in your mouth

Your smoking is unconscious and automatic. Did you ever look down and wonder how that cigarette got in your hand? Raising your awareness and changing patterns are the keys to your success.

routines and patterns

Change your routines and patterns. This is even more true for routines that have to do with smoking.

If you smoke in your car, clean the car inside and out. Remove the lighter and ashtray. Turn on the radio instead of lighting a cigarette. Listen to audio books while you drive. Take a new route to work.

If you smoke after meals, leave the table as soon as you finish eating. Brush your teeth. Keep some after-dinner mints nearby. If you drink coffee, switch from coffee to tea or hot chocolate for a while. Try foods you have never tasted. Sit on the porch. Go for a walk. Go for a drive.

Get the idea? Anything that breaks up your old patterns will make it easier to remember that you quit smoking. Put signs in your kitchen, on your bathroom mirror and at work that say, "I do not smoke."

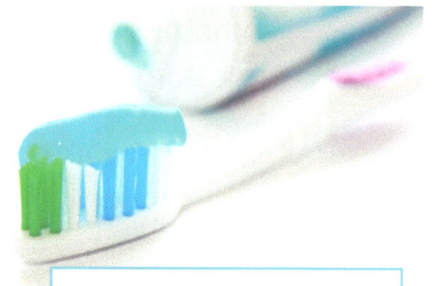

> Write down the when, where and why of every cigarette you smoke for a few weeks before you quit. After you quit, make sure cigarettes are not available at those times or places that you noted.

There are 3 ways to deal with quitting and withdrawal:

1. Quit "**cold turkey**," and wait out the withdrawal symptoms. Symptoms are strongest the first few days and go away over a few weeks. Time is on your side.

2. **Taper down** before you quit so the withdrawal symptoms won't be so intense. To do this, cut down the number of cigarettes you smoke. Go without smoking for part of the day, and gradually increase time between smokes.

3. Use a **nicotine replacement aid**. Starting on your first day without cigarettes. These products help reduce or avoid many of the symptoms of nicotine withdrawal, but they can't make you quit smoking. For best results, use them along with a well-rounded program.

> Use relaxation exercises. Ask those around you to be patient with you.

> It is still very important to set a quit day to stop smoking. You can't become a non-smoker until you do.

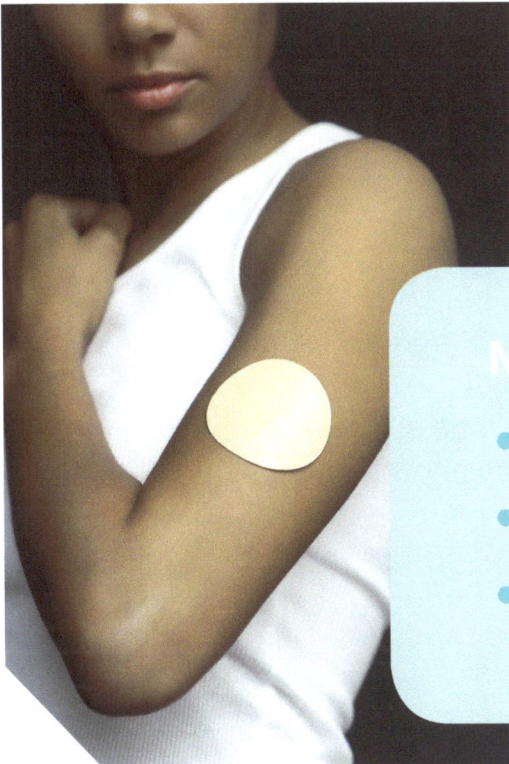

Nicotine Replacement Aids:

- Patch
- Gum
- Nasal spray
- Oral inhaler
- Lozenge
- Prescription drugs

The master plan

Now that you have some good reasons to quit, it's time to make a plan just for you. Fill in the contract on page 20.

- **Choose a quit day.** This is a very important step. Allow enough time to taper your smoking, or get a nicotine replacement aid if you have decided on that route. Choose a day that stands out—like the first day of the week or month. Try to pick a low stress time when there are no other major problems for you to deal with. Plan things to do that day to keep your mind off smoking.

- **Review your reasons for quitting, and list the top 3** on your contract.

- **Commit to a plan.** No matter how good a plan sounds, it can't help you unless you use it. Look over the last few pages, and pick out at least 5 steps that you are willing to use regularly. Write them on your contract.

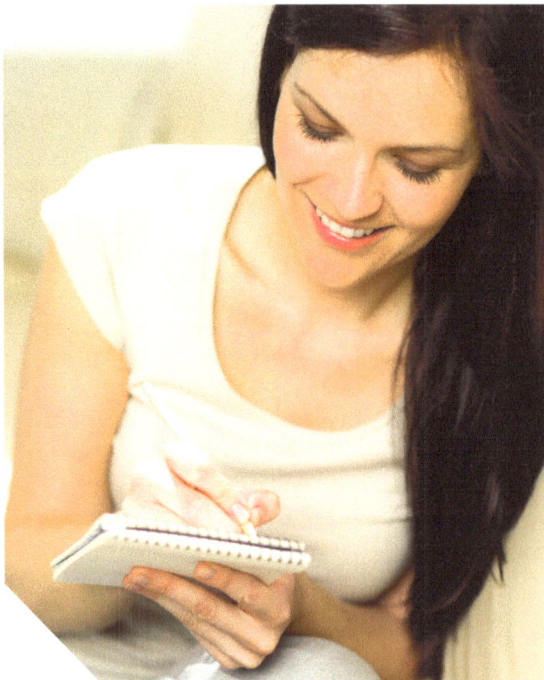

- On your contract, **name 3 people whom you will ask to help you quit.** Tell everyone when you are quitting. Advertise it on quit day by wearing a button or putting up a sign at work. You'll be surprised at how many people will applaud your efforts.

- **List your rewards on your contract.** This is the fun part. Plan rewards for you to collect at certain landmarks in your success. (Review page 12 for ideas.) Even small things like putting a gold star on your calendar every day can make you feel proud of yourself and what you have done.

> Quitting is not easy. It can seem like a long way from the hard part to the good feelings. You will need some payoffs along the way.

Mary, a successful quitter, gave herself a great vacation in the Bahamas as her "final" reward. She was a 2 packs-a-day smoker when she quit. Each day after she quit, she paid the $10.00 she would have spent on smokes to herself and put it in a large jar. After being smoke-free for a year, she decided she had met her goal and counted her money. She had saved almost $3,650! What a time she had—sun, sand, fun and smoke-free.

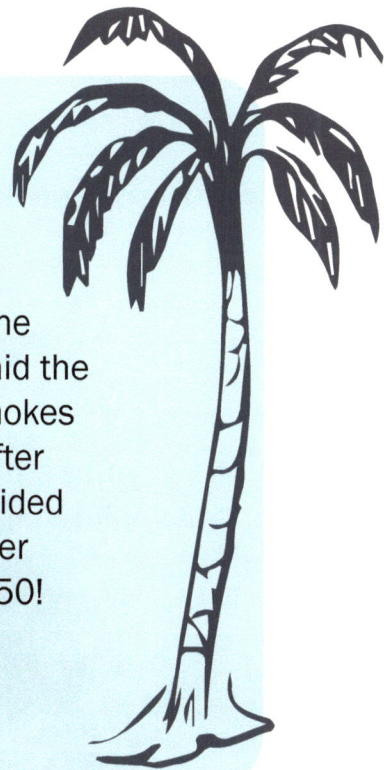

- **Sign your contract.** Make it a serious agreement with yourself. When quit day comes, make it feel special. Throw out all smoking supplies, light a candle, and read your contract aloud. Begin your plan right away.

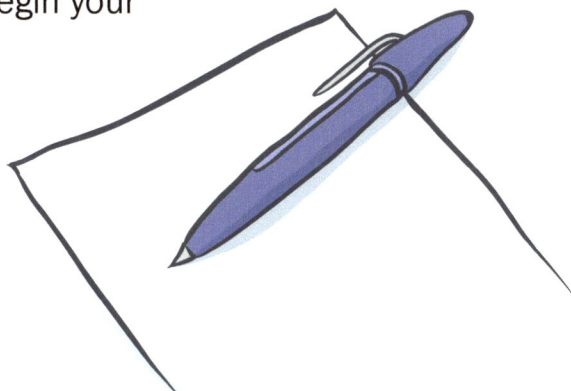

Quit day contract

In order to remain of sound mind and body, I,

_____

(name)

do hereby set forth that I shall quit smoking on

_____

(quit date and renewals)

My most important reasons are:

1.

2.

3.

To answer the urge to smoke, I agree to put the following plan into action:

1.

2.

3.

4.

5.

I have asked the following people for help:

1.

2.

3.

My reward schedule is as follows:

Day 1	Day 4
Day 2	Day 5
Day 3	Day 6

⭐ **Week 1**

Week 2

Week 3

⭐ **1 Month**

2 Months

3 Months

⭐ **6 Months**

⭐ **1 Year**

(make sure the ⭐'s are really special)

Signed _____

(ex-smoker)

Date _____

Witness _____

Other things to help

What about hypnosis, acupuncture and aversion therapy? They have not been widely proven to increase your chances of success, but it is important for you to use whatever you believe will help you to quit for good.

Hypnosis involves making suggestions to your subconscious. It works best if you take conscious steps too.

Acupuncture (use of needles) and acupressure (without the needles) are ancient Chinese therapies to balance the body.

Aversion therapy means creating bad memories associated with smoking. One example is rapid smoking until you feel ill. Do not try rapid smoking unless your doctor says it's safe for you.

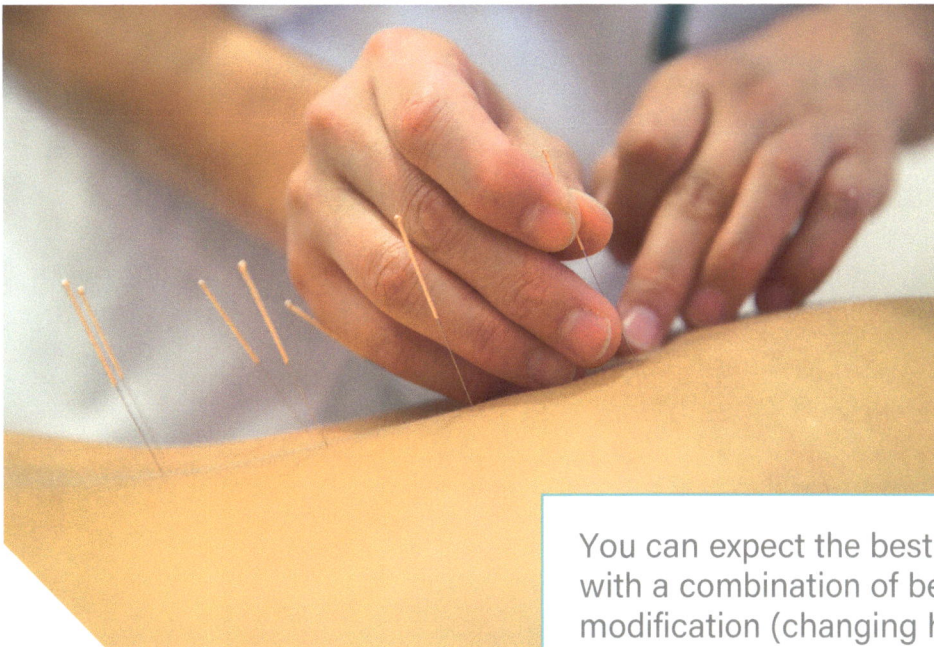

You can expect the best results with a combination of behavior modification (changing habits), education, medicine or nicotine replacement aids, and support programs.

Relapse

Even if you start smoking again, you have taken a giant leap toward quitting for good. You showed the courage to face your problem. If you have slipped back, you now have a chance to find the weak links in your plan and correct them.

Study your slips and your close calls.
Ask yourself these questions:

- Where was I?

- What was I doing?

- Who was I with?

- Where did I get the cigarette?

- How was I feeling?

- Did I have a plan for times like these?

- Did I use my plan?

- What could I do next time to avoid a slip?

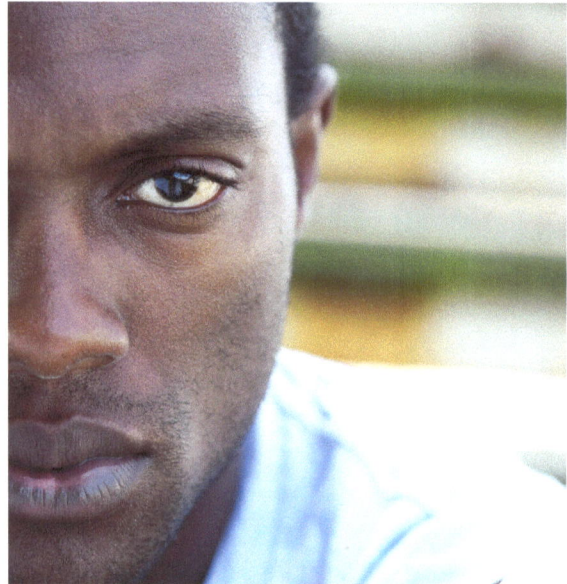

Now you know what didn't work. Revise your plan to include your new approaches or recommit to using the ones you forgot. Don't give up. You're closer than ever. Remember, most successful quitters try 2–6 times before they make it.

Important note: Do not beat up on yourself. **Punishment doesn't work. Forgive yourself.** Think of this effort as a practice run. Set a new quit date. Write your new quit date on the same contract, initial it, and ask your witness to sign it again, too.

Look at your reasons for quitting and the rewards. You can still have them. Reward yourself for trying again. You deserve it.

Where do I go from here?

You're on your way. Your plan is working. It's tempting to believe you don't need your plan anymore, that it's safe to go back to old habits or even have a cigarette once in a while.

Put a "caution" sign on your calendar at 1, 3, 6, 9 months and a year. These are good times to go over your reasons and rewards for quitting.

Be extra careful during very stressful times. Your plan may be enough when you are feeling good, but it may not be in times of crisis or change.

Congratulate yourself every day. Keep rewarding yourself. "Being nice to yourself" will become your new habit and will last long after you stop missing cigarettes.

It only takes one cigarette to start all over again. You are one puff away from 2 packs a day.

On the whole, most smokers are glad to see anyone get free of the habit. A few may still offer you cigarettes. Be ready to say no, and remember your purpose.

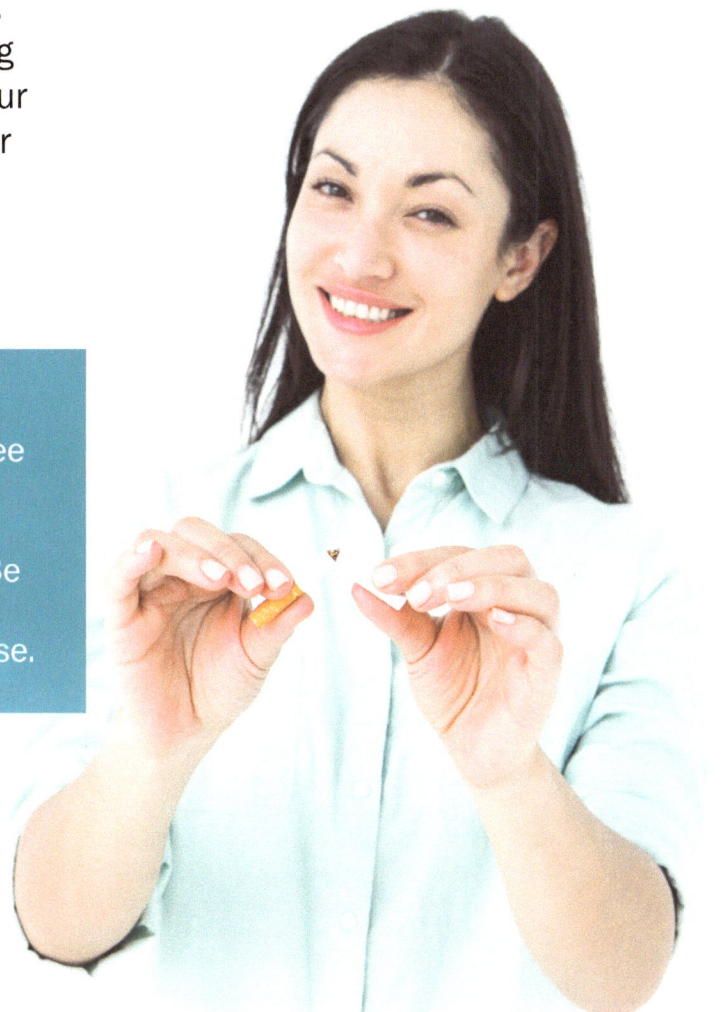

Get help to quit

A **stop-smoking program** may increase your chances of success. Some popular programs include:

- American Lung Association (Freedom From Smoking or Not-on-Tobacco — for teens)

- Smokenders®

- Quit for Life®
  (American Cancer Society)

Search the App Store or Google Play for mobile apps that support your goal of quitting smoking. Many are free. Check with your health care provider, local hospital and employee assistance program about other "quit smoking" programs near you. When checking out programs, be sure to ask about cost, success rates, methods, instructors' training and handouts.

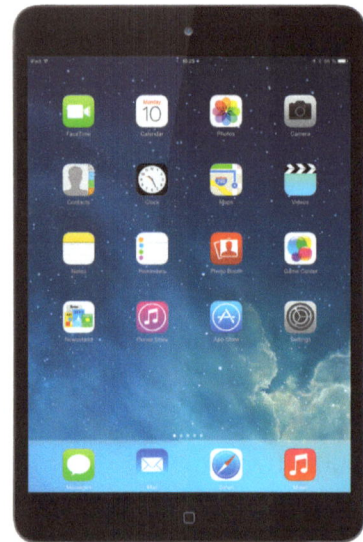

Resources:

American Cancer Society
1-800-ACS-2345
cancer.org

American Heart Association
1-800-AHA-USA1
heart.org

American Lung Association
Freedom From Smoking Program
Not-on-Tobacco (teens)
1-800-LUNG-USA
lung.org

National Cancer Institute
1-800-4-CANCER
cancer.gov

Notes:

Order this book from :

PRITCHETT & HULL ASSOCIATES, INC.
3440 OAKCLIFF RD NE STE 126
ATLANTA GA 30340-3006

or call toll free: **800-241-4925**

ISBN #978-1-943234-06-6

2018 Edition
Published and distributed by:
Pritchett & Hull Associates, Inc.

Printed in the U.S.A.

www.ingramcontent.com/pod-product-compliance
Lightning Source LLC
Chambersburg PA
CBHW060857270326
41934CB00003B/184